YOGA & HEALTH
with Mary Rose Doorly

GILL AND MACMILLAN
and
RADIO TELEFÍS ÉIREANN

Published by
Gill and Macmillan Ltd
Goldenbridge
Dublin 8
and
Radio Telefís Éireann
Donnybrook
Dublin 4
© Mary Rose Doorly 1990
0 7171 1823 1
Edited by Roberta Reeners
Designed by Design Image, Dublin
Line illustrations by Cathy Henderson
Colour origination by Kulor Centre Ltd
Printed by Criterion Press, Dublin

ACKNOWLEDGMENTS

I wish to thank the following for their kind help and assistance when this book was in preparation.
For clothing: Airwave, Pia Bang, Arnott's Sports Department, Puma and Benetton.
For the food shots: Gallery 22.
MRD

CONTENTS

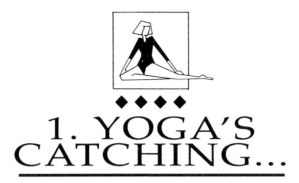

◆ ◆ ◆ ◆
1. YOGA'S CATCHING...

Welcome to a really different approach to exercise. I promise I'm not going to talk about pain, only pleasure.

Why has Yoga made such a huge comeback recently? Why are people turning back to Yoga and stretch exercises as though they were completely new inventions? If you are a follower of the Yoga slot on 'Live at 3', you are already converted, or reconverted to the idea of an effortless and enjoyable way of getting totally fit.

So many of the people I know who have kept up their Yoga over the years remain calm and relaxed. What's more, they have remained fit; and in perfect shape too. Meeting them is encountering living proof. Why? Because Yoga is something you can live with - something which fits so easily into your daily lifestyle that you can't resist it - something which gives you fitness, relaxation, weight loss and complete health, almost by default.

Take weight loss, for example. You can't do Yoga for any length of time without feeling the benefits. Before long, you become so much more aware of your own body, and the pleasure of moving through stretching and balancing sequences, that you gain self discipline, self esteem and, above all, self control. Before long, you gain the motivation to improve your life in a permanent and positive way. With Yoga ... you won't know yourself.

We are used to thinking that terms such as 'selfish', 'self centred', 'self interested' are used to describe unkind, ungenerous individuals. I believe the opposite - provided, of course, that your individuality includes something as positive as Yoga. If you cannot be selfish once in a while, if you don't believe you deserve a slice of relaxation and personal fitness, then you can hardly expect to be fully in control. Self interest gives you motivation.

The first responsibility of any human being is to their own sanity, health and physical welfare. Anyone who neglects that duty of living a full, enjoyable and healthy life will risk becoming a burden on themselves or others. So why not spoil yourself on Yoga? It's one of the most 'selfish' and worthwhile things you can ever do. You deserve it.

◆ ◆ ◆ ◆
New Yoga

Over the past number of years, I have been developing completely new Yoga routines which are easy to follow and so enjoyable to carry out at home that they become second nature. That was always the secret with Yoga, that you could keep it up forever. You become a fan. It's like a lifelong addiction. Once you get involved in Yoga, you never let go; you'll always insist on getting your quota of peaceful exercise, at least once every day.

What I have done with Yoga is to take it a step further. By arranging these 2000-year-old Yoga poses or *asanas* in sequences which take no longer than three to five minutes each, I have structured them into a continuous and planned course of movements. By following an easily remembered sequence of movements, you will be inclined to follow your routine more regularly and adopt Yoga as part of your day. Each sequence is designed to deal with a specific area of the body and intended for weight control, relaxation and overall muscle toning. Above all, these *asanas* are intended to increase flexibility, strength and energy.

The idea for sequence Yoga came from one of the oldest Yoga concepts - the Salute to the Sun - which you will find in this book. Many people I know have enjoyed doing this morning stretch sequence so much over the years that they began to ask me if there were any other sequences I could show them. So I began to work on the idea of new sequences, incorporating all the disparate elements of a Yoga session into easily manageable routines.

What this New Yoga does, above all else, is to create lovely, flowing movements from one pose into the next. The idea is to establish a continuous progression of slow-motion exercise from which you will receive great benefits all round.

◆ ◆ ◆ ◆
How to use this book

Each chapter in this book contains one sequence. Excluding the final chapter which deals with chair exercises, there are seven chapters and seven sequences - one for each day of the week. In addition to the written instructions and the photographs showing you how to carry out each sequence, you will see each entire sequence described from beginning to end in graphics.

The first and most important thing to do before any new exercise programme is to consult your doctor. For anyone over the age of thirty-five, this is vital. Once you have taken your doctor's advice, you can be certain that your individual concerns are being taken care of and that your routine is entirely safe.

◆ ◆ ◆ ◆
How to begin

For Yoga, one thing you need is a warm, comfortable environment, free from intrusion and disturbance. You also need loose, comfortable clothes, a mat or a towel to lie on and perhaps one or two cushions strategically placed to add comfort to the spine or the neck. Most important of all is that you choose a certain time (twenty or thirty minutes each day) which is guaranteed to be yours, on your own. If you like, you can put on some soft music while you go through the sequence.

Remember!

- Wear loose, comfortable clothing. Remove the shoes.
- Always exercise before mealtimes.
- There should be no pain, just a gentle stretch.
- If you feel pain, move out of the pose until it is more comfortable.
- If you are pregnant, you should not do this or any exercise routine without checking with your gynaecologist. Avoid all abdominal exercises.

- If you have a back or neck problem, suffer from rheumatism, arthritis or have a heart complaint, you should make sure to check with your doctor before starting these exercises.

- With all of the sequences, make sure that you carry on breathing rhythmically. As you become more familiar with the sequences, you may like to try the deeper breathing techniques described in Chapter 7.

- To derive maximum benefit from these sequences, ensure that the progression from each pose to the next is carried out as slowly and as gracefully as possible. This also increases the enjoyment of Yoga.

◆ ◆ ◆ ◆
THE WAVE SEQUENCE

The Wave Sequence is a lovely series of poses which gives great flexibility and tone to the waist, legs and back. You will also find it very effective in firming the stomach and bottom. As with all Yoga *asanas*, you can make this sequence as easy or as hard as you wish by reducing or increasing the stretch. It's up to you to decide how far you want to stretch and how long you wish to hold for. If you have difficulty sitting on your heels, then raise your weight off your heels by kneeling up.

1. Sit on your heels. Back tall and shoulders down. Without rounding the back, clasp your hands together. Keeping the arms straight, raise them up behind your back.

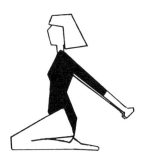

2. Keeping the hands in the clasped position, slowly begin to bend the body forward. If you can bring your head down onto the floor ... well done! If not, don't worry and don't strain. Just go as far as you can. You'll be able to place your head on the floor if you lift your weight off your heels. Hold for 3. Slowly bring the body back to the sitting position and unclasp the hands.

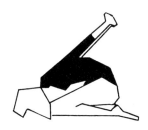

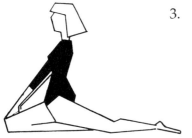

3. Remain sitting on your heels and stretch your left leg out behind you. Place both hands on your right knee. If you are losing your balance, then put your hands on the floor on either side of your knee. Stretch your body up as tall as you can. Hold for 3.

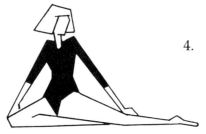

4. Bring your left hand around and, turning to the side, place it on your outstretched leg. You should feel a lovely stretch in the waist. Hold for 3.

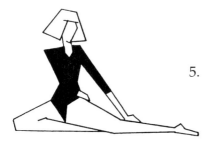

5. Now bring your right hand around and place it on your waist. Hold for 3.

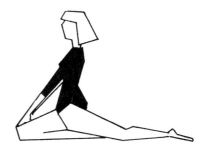

6. Smoothly return both hands around to the front and place them on your right knee. Remain kneeling. Keeping the left leg out, stretch the body up as tall as you can. Hold for 3.

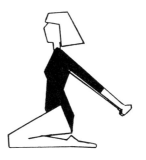

7. Return your left leg to its original position beside the right knee. Clasp the hands together behind the back and raise them up as much as you can, comfortably. (See position 1.) Make sure you don't round the shoulders. Hold for 3.

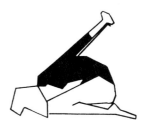

8. Keep your hands joined as you bend the body forward onto the floor. If you can't place your head on the floor while sitting on the heels, then lift your weight off your heels until you can comfortably rest your head on the floor. Hold for 3. Because this part of the sequence is so relaxing, you may prefer to stay in this position for longer.

*Repeat the entire sequence 5 times, alternating the right and left leg each time. As it becomes easier to do, you may wish to increase the hold to a slow count of 5 or even 10.

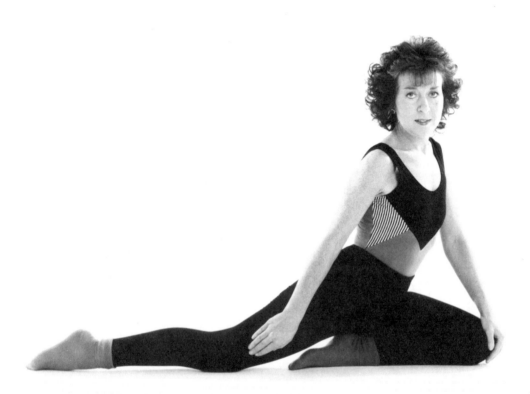

▲ *Feel a lovely stretch along your waist as you slowly twist around and reach back with your arm (Position 4).*

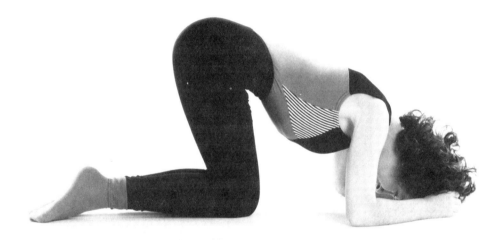

▲ *If you find it difficult to raise your hands behind you in the kneeling pose, you may prefer to try this variation (Position 8).*

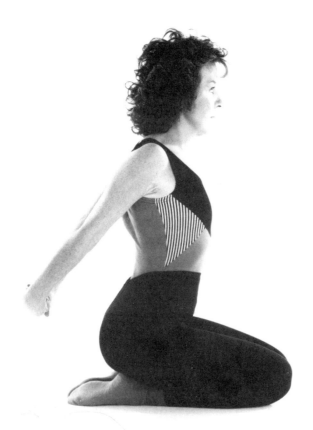

▲ *Make sure to keep your back straight in this position. This one is excellent for posture (Positions 1 and 7).*

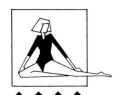

2. YOU AND YOUR ENVIRONMENT

Believe it or not, they say that only a very small percentage of people in this world actually make free choices. The rest of us are pushed, cajoled and led by decisions made elsewhere. Whether we like it or not, we cannot resist the overt or more subliminal pressures placed upon us by advertising, by fashion, by the trends of our environment. How much real choice do we have?

The pressures from our choices come in a variety of ways - in the supermarket, from the media (mainly from TV) and from our own friends. Luckily, in the past few years, consumers have begun to lash back with their own demands for healthy food and a healthy environment. Long may it last!

But what about your own personal environment? How free are we to move in our own living space? One of the most valuable fashions to come up in the past few decades is the trend towards exercise and personal fitness, underlining the huge benefits which we derive from a healthy lifestyle. Exercise is the one certain way in which we can really defy all pressures. And how can we expect to take a more active role in our environment generally if we don't practise that same control over our own limited choices? Yoga is one of your free choices. Why not take it?

◆ ◆ ◆
Confined Bodies

One of the most telling results of the world we live in is the area of stress and tension (see Chapter 7). So much of our lifestyle confines us to a poor range of movements, manifesting itself in poor posture and inadequate relaxation. Our bodies can easily reflect the state of our surroundings. What we have to remember is that comfortable homes don't always mean comfortable bodies.

Unless we take an active part in the maintenance of our own bodies with Yoga or other forms of exercise, we yield only too easily to the pressures around us. Round shoulders, tense necks, backache and tension in the body can often be the results of the way we fit into our lifestyle. A bad fit, maybe.

One of the important things to remember about posture is that it not only reflects our mood and our personality; it also reflects how we perceive ourselves. Posture is a deep thing, not just something superficial which can be adjusted on the spot.

The postural muscles in the body are not positioned on the surface. They are not the muscles we use for activities like running. Instead, the postural muscles, the muscles that hold your back straight and your head high while you are stationary, are positioned closer to the skeletal structure. They are mainly hidden and cannot easily be felt under the skin.

All the more reason to manage your body in such a way that it adopts a superior posture. It will reflect your positive personality and your self awareness. This is one of the main benefits of practising Yoga. Unlike cardiovascular exercise (any activity which makes your heart beat faster), very necessary in its own right, Yoga works most effectively on that range of muscles which control the posture. After Yoga sequences such as you'll find in this book, your posture will improve automatically and the postural muscles will remember their proper role, to carry the body efficiently.

◆ ◆ ◆
Scientific

In the eighties, there was a sudden emphasis on science in exercise. Every muscle movement involved in training had to be studied, measured and explained. Cardiovascular endurance was pitched against flexibility and stretch movements. It seemed like a contest between followers of various fitness programmes. As a result of all this scientific interest, physiotherapists and kineaseologists have made major advances in eliminating the dangers of exercise, ensuring that exercise programmes have become much safer.

With this increasing emphasis placed on cardiovascular fitness, however, people began to take up aerobics almost to the exclusion of stretch and flexibility programmes. Each new aerobic programme claimed to be the only way to get fit and to lose weight, quite unjustifiably pushing Yoga and other valuable routines aside. There is no doubt that cardiovascular fitness is essential (see Chapter 6) but Yoga, and especially this newly-arranged sequence Yoga, provides the proper base for complete fitness.

For many people, unable to deal with the unreasonable effort demanded by heavy-duty cardiovascular training, many aerobic routines never succeeded because they were that bit too tough. The sheer effort can be discouraging in itself and lead to a massive fall-off rate. Nothing will put you off exercise as quickly as fatigue. The drop-out rate from Yoga is far lower because it works on the principle of a lifetime routine. It's not just for a short burst. For so many people, Yoga is not just the perfect compromise, but also the most prolonged and enjoyable workout of all.

Why exercise? It is vital to make up your mind and have a good reason for exercising. It's a big mistake to exercise just to fit into the slender formula which the media hold out for us to follow. Why imitate? Why not do it just for yourself? Why not do it to feel comfortable with yourself and to feel that wonderful control over your personal environment?

◆ ◆ ◆ ◆
THE CAT SEQUENCE

The Cat Sequence will greatly improve the strength, flexibility and posture of the back. The poses are also extremely effective in firming up the bottom, hips and thighs.

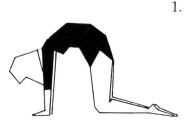

1. Kneel down on the floor, on your hands and knees. Place the hands directly beneath your shoulders. Arch your back up as high as you can ... much like a cat having a good stretch. Don't bend your arms and, to exercise the tummy, pull in the abdomen as much as possible. Hold for 3.

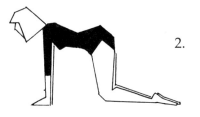

2. Sink the back down and raise your head. Make sure that you keep the arms straight. Hold for 3.

3. Raise the right knee and bring it in as close as possible to your head. Keep the right foot off the floor.

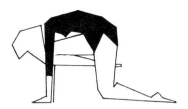

4. Smoothly and with control, lift the right leg into the air behind you. Lift it as high as you can without straining ... mind that back! Hold for 3.

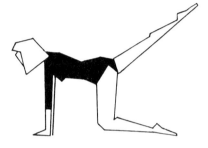

5. Bend the right knee and bring your foot in towards your back. Flex the foot. Don't let your knee sink down. Hold for 3.

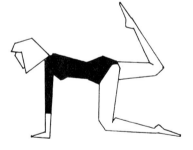

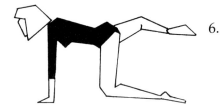

6.   Keeping your right knee bent, slowly bring your right leg out to the side. Point the toe and keep the leg in the raised position. Hold for 3.

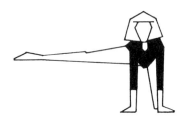

7.   Gradually straighten out your right leg to the side and hold in the raised position. You'll find this pose a little tougher to do. Do your best. Just think of those saddle bags disappearing! Hold for 3.

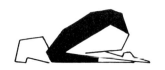

8.   Sit down on your heels to do one of my favourite poses. Gently bend over and place your head on the floor in front of your knees. Let your hands lie loosely along either side of your thighs on the floor. If you have difficulty in sitting on your heels, then come forward until you can manage the pose more comfortably. Hold for 3 or, since it's an enjoyable pose, for as long as you wish.

* Repeat the entire sequence 5 times with both legs. As the Cat becomes easier to do, you may like to increase the hold up to 5 or even 10.

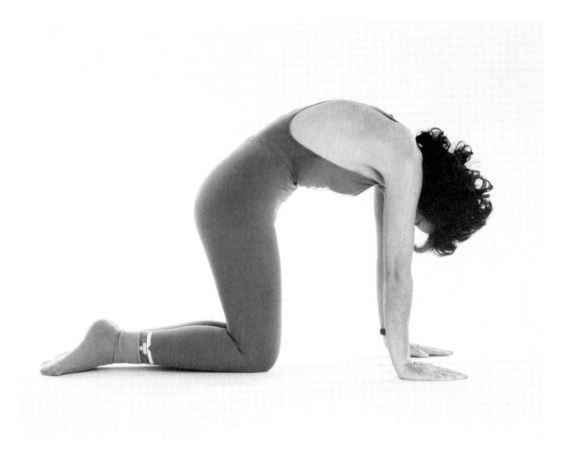

▲ *Arch the back as high as you can ... much like a cat having a good stretch (Position 1).*

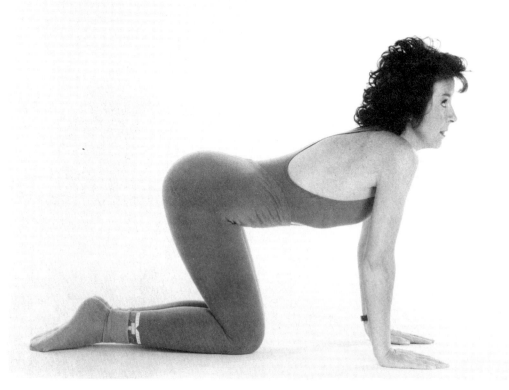

▲ *Move slowly and allow the small of the back to sink down (Position 2).*

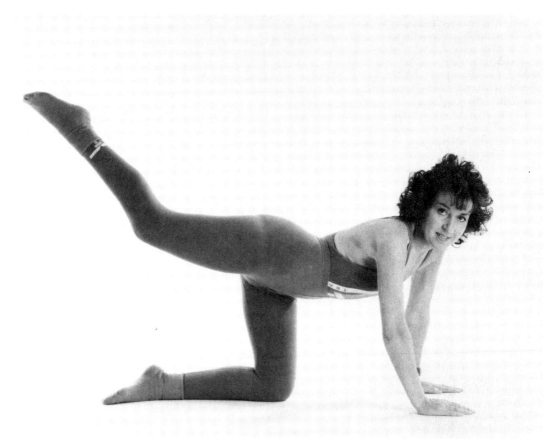

▲ *Stretch the leg right up behind you - don't strain (Position 4).*

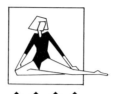

♦ ♦ ♦ ♦
3. LOSE WEIGHT WITH NEW YOGA

♦ ♦ ♦ ♦
The Battle

You've tried everything. Again and again, you've faced the challenge. You've brought the latest weight loss plan. Inspired by the latest promises, you've tried yet another diet. The last resort, you say. This better work.

Sometimes it does work. You lose a few inches - a few pounds disappear miraculously from the critical areas: the thighs, the tummy, the waist ... that bottom. But then, lo and behold, you come back to square one again. You abandon that latest weight loss plan. In despair, you console yourself with ... guess what? Food. It's like a complete circle.

Why are your efforts failing? Why is that success in weight loss so elusive? Why is it that, every time you get anywhere and you just begin to fit back into your size twelve clothes, the whole thing falls apart again, you lose the initiative and bow out? If anything, you might as well have not done it at all, because now you feel demoralised into the bargain. You give up hope.

♦ ♦ ♦ ♦
Failure vs Success

What is it about failure that's so close to success? When it comes to weight loss, we have nobody to blame but ourselves. Nobody else can do it for us. That's what makes it so bad. If only we could pay somebody to take away the problem - and the excess weight. But that's it. You buy the diet books, the latest exercise video, the magic cures (the diet industry in the USA is now put at $30 billion per annum), anything but own up to the simple reality that it's entirely your problem. It's personal.

In fact it's so personal that you don't even want to talk about it. For most overweight people, it's a lonely problem, fighting with an enemy that doesn't ever come out into the open. You can't stop eating. You have to live. It's not like drinking alcohol where you can make yourself stay out of bars, or like gambling where you can tell yourself to steer clear of the betting shops. Food is a must. That's why it's so difficult.

As well as that, we have now turned food into a culture, a social interaction. We communicate with food. We cook to celebrate, to impress, to make friends. Food is part of giving and accepting hospitality. Food is entertainment. You can't say no.

◆ ◆ ◆
Overweight experts

Ever since I began working with exercise and encouraging overweight people, the most fascinating thing I have discovered is that the overweight person already knows everything about weight loss. They know every diet. Every slimming programme has passed through their hands. Many of the people I have known could even reel off the exact order in which diet books came out. They never miss anything. Overweight people, in my experience, are usually the greatest experts on obesity. They usually know all about cellulite, about calories, fibre diets, fruit diets. They've tried the appetite inhibitors, the slimming tablets and the food replacement drinks. They know about skipping meals, about fasting, even the equal and opposite dangers of anorexia nervosa. They know all the common sense advice about dieting, like eating off a smaller plate, chewing an apple half an hour before a meal, never shopping on an empty stomach.

If you are overweight, you will also know all about exercise. 'I've tried aerobics - it doesn't work for me,' you hear yourself say. 'I've tried joining a gym, I've tried running, jazz ballet, you name it. Nothing works!' But isn't there some inbuilt contradiction there? Trying isn't enough. You need something more permanent. Only a permanent plan will give you permanent results.

◆ ◆ ◆ ◆
Where are you going wrong?

So what is the answer? Why does that perfect resolve and will power always fail? The truth is that obesity and overweight problems are more than just a matter of calories in and calories out. What is now being established is that obesity is far more a personality problem. It has to do with motivation, getting to grips with the idea of developing a new attitude and a new lifestyle.

Confronting the problem is the first and hardest part of all. Acknowledging the fact that you are overweight, that it greatly affects not only your health and the length of your life but also your personal happiness as well, is the most difficult stage to get over. You have to stop deluding yourself that you look well, that you look slimmer in a dark outfit and that because nobody talks about it, you're getting away with it. You have to dismiss the compliments, the endearments and the kind words of relatives and friends who say you're looking well.

Owning up to the facts is hard. If you want permanent results, it's the only way. The first thing you should do is get a complete medical check-up. Once you get the news about your blood pressure, the strain on your heart, on your back, on your digestive system, and the fact that you are putting your entire well-being at risk, you'll get that vital start, the primary motivation.

◆ ◆ ◆ ◆
The Overweight Factors

There are many different factors involved in the overweight problem. It's not just a matter of food or exercise. Let's list the factors.

1. Hereditary Factors

If your parents or grandparents were overweight, then there may be a greater likelihood that you will be the same. But that doesn't mean you can do nothing about it. Even more reason for you to break the chain. Quite apart from these inherited genes, we also inherit many habits and traditions. For instance, if the mother places an emphasis on cakes and sweet things, the children will be more than willing to take up that ideology of the sweet tooth.

One overweight person put it very succinctly to me when she said that mothers like to surround themselves with eaters, if only to justify their own eating habits. So don't spoil the children. You might be spoiling yourself.

2.   Metabolism

It's just not fair, you will say. The well-established fact is that no two people are the same, and the rate at which each one of us metabolises food varies enormously. Why me, you ask. Why does the same sized doughnut reek havoc on the waist of one person, where it is burned up in pure activity with another?

Blame it on evolution. In another era, back in the days when food was scarce, the overweight tendency was an innate and valuable storage system. The body of a survivor, you could say. Now, in different circumstances, that metabolism seems like a curse. And there is little we can do about it, except that it is proven that exercise increases the rate at which you metabolise up to hours after your workout, particularly if you raise the heart rate and make the exercise cardiovascular. That's where the good brisk walk comes in.

3.   Occupational Factors

The nature of your work can have a direct influence on your weight. I've talked to everybody from politicians to housewives, all of them describing food as an absolute hazard - almost like a trap door waiting for them to fall into. The busy man or woman going to receptions, business lunches and working late at night will develop erratic eating habits where food and the choice of food is taken completely out of their hands.

If, for instance, your occupation requires you to spend long hours catering or dealing with food (the obvious example might be the role of a mother or father feeding a gang of children), you'll be faced with the same difficulties. Can you imagine working in a cake shop and not eating cakes? Or working in an office where your colleagues have established a round system of cream slices? Now at last it's become acceptable and even trendy to say 'no' to your cholesterol fetish.

It's important to analyse clearly your particular occupation and its hazards.

4. Food Intake

Obviously, the nature of the food you consume will have a huge bearing on your weight. Alcohol, fats and sugars are some of the main culprits which we will be discussing later in the book. But it is important not to isolate food as the only factor involved in obesity.

There are a variety of medical problems which can also affect your weight. Therefore it is very important to go for that full check-up and discuss any new diet or exercise programmes with your doctor.

5. Social Factors

Like it or not, the average person is greatly influenced by the society around them. When you piece together the set of influences, the range of choices in the supermarket, the TV ads, the fads in food and the constant pressures to fit into the shapely image idealised by the media, we are actually left with very little choice in our lives.

Overweight problems are very often the result of this massive pressure from all areas of your environment, leading to a situation where you have virtually handed over control of your own mind and body. You must ask yourself whether your overweight problem is a matter of personal mismanagement.

The way to tackle this management problem seriously is to examine and confront your situation and your own eating patterns, something we'll be going into in the next chapter.

♦ ♦ ♦ ♦
THE BRIDGE SEQUENCE

This sequence is specifically designed to work on the stomach muscles. Very few of our daily movements have any effect on the abdominal muscles, which makes it vital to work on that area every day. With this sequence, you exercise all the abdominal muscles, beginning by working on the middle and lower tummy, right through to the obliques. The stretching effect throughout this movement is amplified by keeping the stomach pulled in.

Remember also that this sequence will greatly improve the condition of your back in the process, because of the important role the abdominal muscles play in supporting the spine.

1. Lie on your back. Knees bent. Feet in as close to the bottom as possible. Raise your hips up from the floor and keep them raised until position 8. Make sure you don't strain your back by lifting too high. Hands on the floor. Pull the tummy muscles in as tightly as possible. Hold for 3. Relax the stomach muscles and tighten again 3 times.

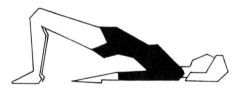

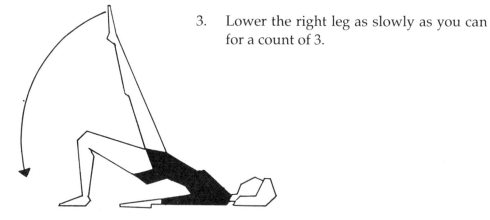

2. Straighten out the right leg. Raise into the air for 3. Keep the hips up. Hold for 3.

3. Lower the right leg as slowly as you can for a count of 3.

4. Raise the left leg.

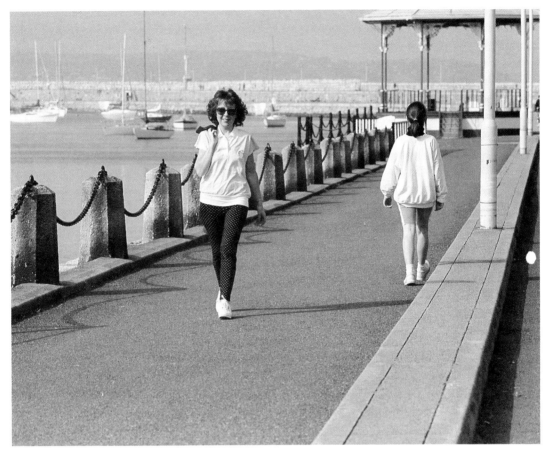

▲ *Walking a mile is as good as running a mile.*

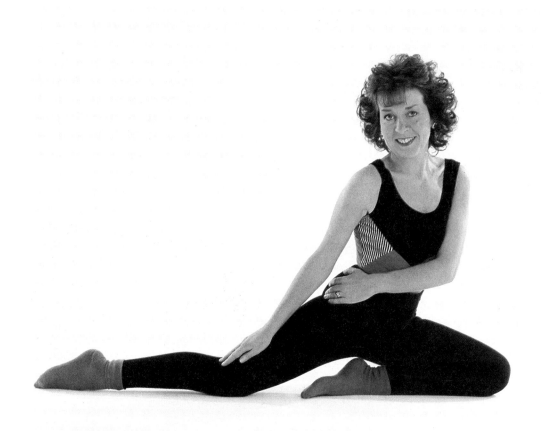

▲ *Once you get a taste for Yoga, you never let go (The Wave Sequence).*

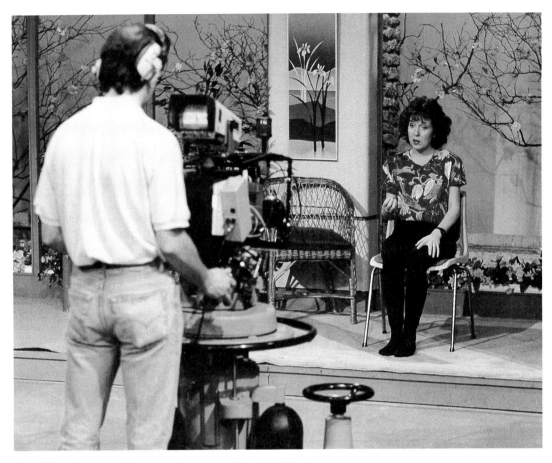

▲ *'They're not sultanas or bananas, Derek. They're asanas.*
(Yoga on the 'Live at 3' set)

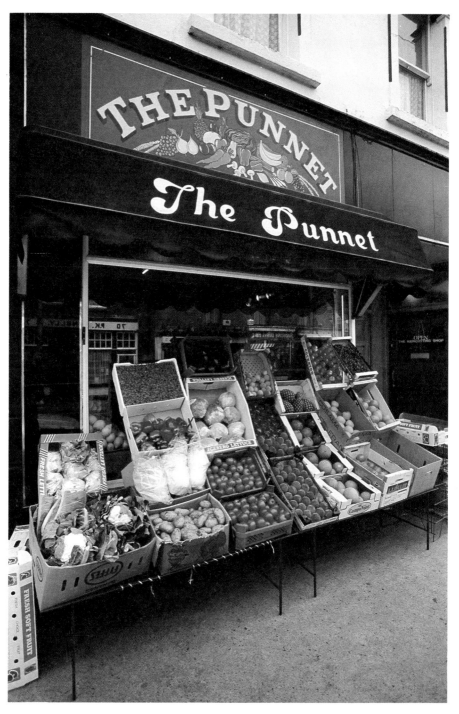

▲ *Open a nutritious account with your local greengrocer.*

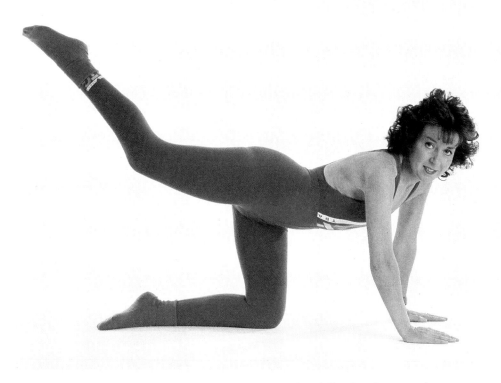

▲ *Yoga works on the principle of a lifetime routine (The Cat Sequence).*

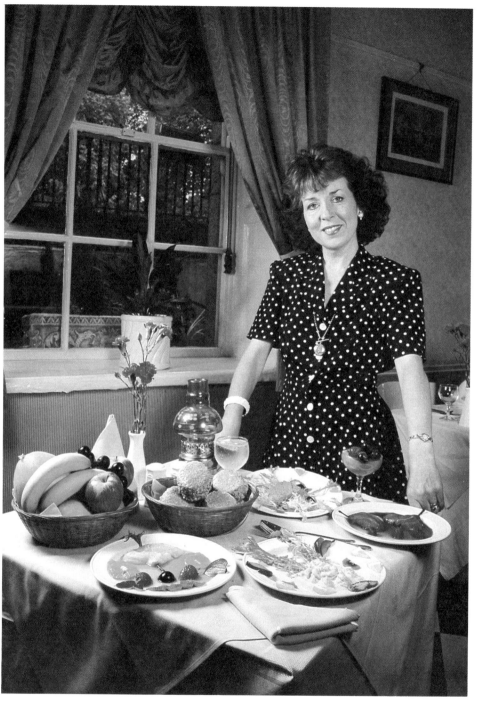

▲ *Everything here is low in cholesterol ... including the carnations.*

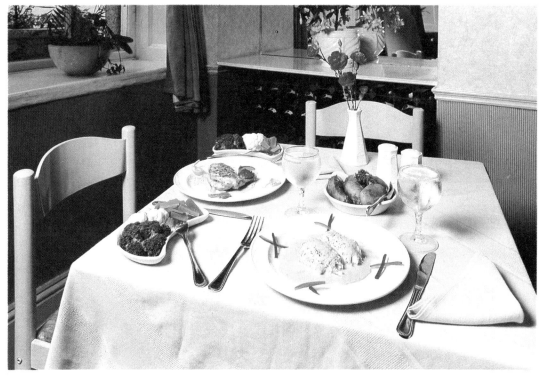

▲ *Forget dieting. Develop an appetite for light food and exercise.*

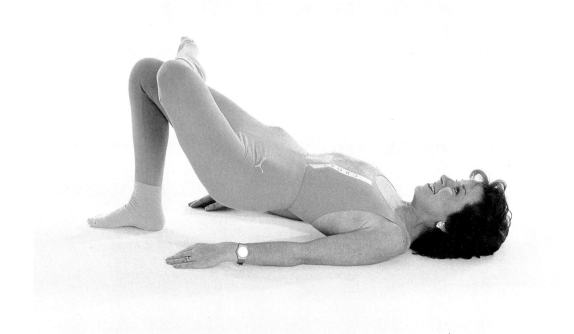

▲ *Try a different sequence every day (The Bridge Sequence).*

5. Lower that leg as slowly as you can for a count of 3.

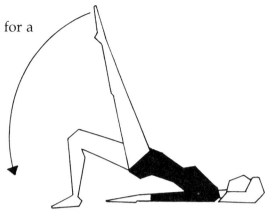

6. Keeping the hips raised, bend the right leg and place the right foot on top of the left knee. Push the left knee out and down towards the floor for an inner thigh stretch. Hold for 3.

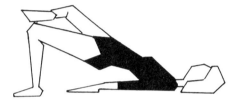

7. Raise the left leg and repeat with the left foot on the right knee this time. Hold for 3.

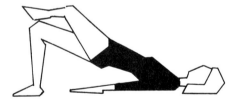

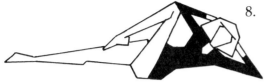

8. Lower the hips onto the floor slowly. Raise the left knee to meet the right elbow. Keep the right leg outstretched and an inch or so off the floor. Hold for 3.

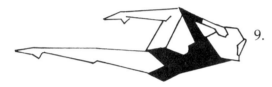

9. Raise the right knee to meet the left elbow. Hold for 3.

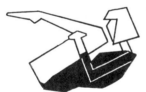

10. Hug both knees into the chest and raise your head up towards the knees. Hold for 3.

    Lie on the floor, close your eyes and relax completely.

* Repeat the entire sequence 5 times. As it become easier to do, you can increase the hold for a slow count of 5 or even up to 10.

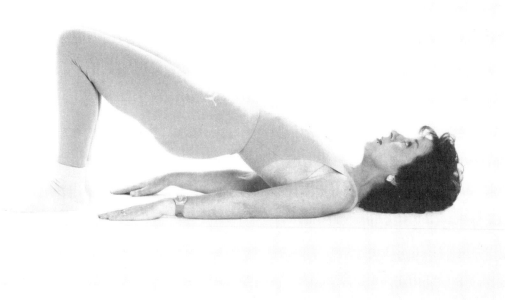

▲ *Concentrate on pulling your tummy in as tightly as you can in this raised position (Position 1).*

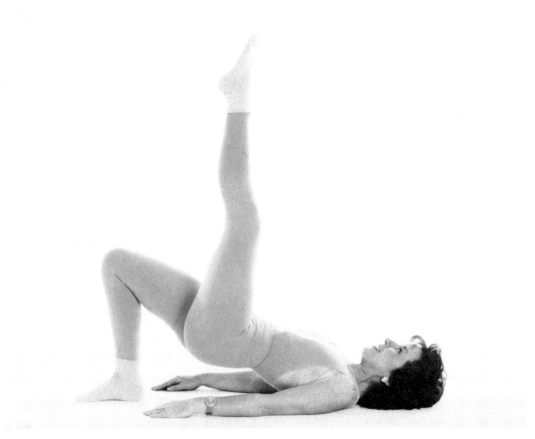

▲ *Raise your leg, pointing the toe upwards (Position 4).*

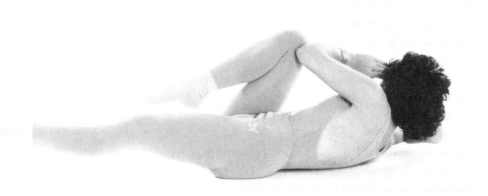

▲ *Place your left elbow on your right knee and stretch your left leg out (Position 9).*

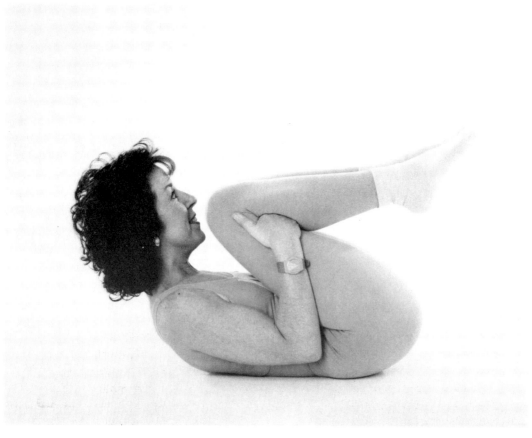

▲ *Hugging your knees into your chest gives great relief to an aching back (Position 10).*

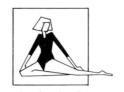

◆ ◆ ◆ ◆
4. PSYCHING UP FOR SUCCESS

◆ ◆ ◆ ◆
A New Start

You may not believe it, but it is perfectly possible that you will soon get your weight under control for good. Even if you have failed before and tried many diets that haven't worked for you, don't worry - you still have one good chance left. This time you'll do it right. This time you won't be going for overnight success but a process of firm, level-headed and unspectacular change.

This time, it's for good. Turning over a new leaf always sounds like a miracle. The only miracle you can bank on is a slow miracle. You have to turn over that new leaf every day, not just one day. Every day of your life is a tiny new start.

The most important discovery about weight control in the past few year is that diets generally don't work. New lifestyles do. The latest concept in weight loss which is supported by many experts in the field is that we must move away from the idea of a one-day wonder and switch on to this new lifestyle approach. Something that will last. You want to be able to look back in a while and say: 'I used to eat that kind of thing... I used to buy those doughnuts... I used to go for cream, cheesecake, pizza ... now my tastebuds are enjoying new, healthier foods.'

The first thing you have to do is to psyche yourself up. Follow these points and you'll gain the right momentum.

- Be positive. Believe you can gain control of your weight.
- Don't expect immediate success. Weight disappears the same way as you put it on - *slowly.*

- Demystify food. Stop treating food as an escape from life. Find other interests. Treat food as fuel for a good life.

- Deal with stress. If your life is under great stress, you may be using food as a consolation. We tend to resort to food when we feel badly, under pressure or in a state of anxiety. Equally, we tend to reward ourselves with food when we feel good, saying: 'To hell with it, I feel great. I'll have a bar of chocolate.' Stress can knock the best intentions off course.

- Avoid the weighing scales. They are not an accurate measure of success. Only weigh yourself occasionally when you already feel successful.

- Give yourself time to adjust. You are moving into a brand new life.

- Be honest. You can't fool yourself.

◆◆◆◆
Confront Yourself

Many of the world's leading health experts are now blaming the lack of success in dieting on the fact that it is such a stop-start process; the revolving door syndrome. If you have failed at dieting before, you will only too easily place yourself in that category again, endlessly going around the revolving door getting nowhere, neither inside or outside the building. What you end up with is a growing feeling of despair, nothing else.

What we are interested in from now on is a growing feeling of success, nothing else.

Psychologists and weight specialists are now talking about the natural period of readjustment - a critical phase of withdrawal followed by a slow phase of rebuilding, almost brick by brick. They talk about a process which can in some cases take several years, a process which is like any other stage of life, like the teenage years or mid life. The latest scientific concept of weight loss (permanent weight loss) is the idea of a life cycle, a slow revolution of radical new principles of food and exercise. It's all a bit like saving for a house.

Hang on a minute! Here is where you gasp and say: 'I don't want this to take ten years!' But just think about it: if you fail to take this permanent approach, you'll end up in ten years' time right back where you started, an eternal dieter. This is where you need to confront yourself and call for action.

◆ ◆ ◆ ◆
Good Reasons

To whip up any degree of motivation and self belief, you have to want something badly. Agreed? You have to want it so badly that you would change your life for it. This is where you confront yourself and examine the precise reasons why you want to lose weight.

1. Look good. (You want to look young and energetic. You realise that weight is making you look heavy and slow.)

2. Feel energetic and lead a healthy, active life. (You want to avoid all the associated health problems like high blood pressure, heart irregularities, digestive disorders and many other risks.)

3. Fit into normal clothes. (You are fed up with the constant reminder that your wardrobe is designed for somebody else.)

4. Gain self esteem. (You are fed up lying to yourself, getting depressed about your weight and despairing about lack of success.)

Vanity can actually turn out to be one of the best motives in the world. If it gets you out of the food trap, what's wrong with loving yourself, feeling important ... a bit of narcissism won't go astray. Call it self respect.

◆ ◆ ◆ ◆
Downfalls of Dieting

- Dieting doesn't alter long-term eating patterns.
- Dieting upsets your internal balance of water and minerals.
- Dieting can lead to low blood pressure, leaving you weak, with heart irregularities.

- Dieting can make you gain weight. While you're on a diet, your body learns to adapt to fewer calories, thereby using energy from food more efficiently. Once you give up the diet, you put on weight faster because your body has learned to store any excess.

- Dieting plays with your emotions. The on-off cycle of dieting reeks havoc on your confidence.

◆ ◆ ◆ ◆
Sizing up your weight

First things first. Before you make the new start, you need to know exactly where you are on the scale of body weight versus height. The scale below will give you an indication of whether your weight is healthy or not in relation to your size. This is a new scientific index developed by Canadian health specialists.

Instructions for the Body Mass Index

Mark an X at your height on scale A.

Mark an X at your weight on scale B.

Draw a line to join the two Xs.

Extend this line to scale C to find where you are on the BMI.

Exceptions: this index is only accurate for people with stable weight, aged between 20 and 65.

Example:

Bridget is 5ft 4 inches tall and weighs 9 stone

Her BMI is just above 21.

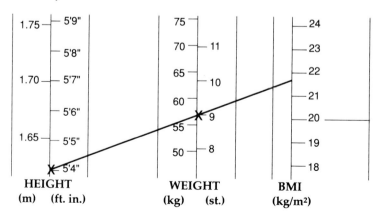

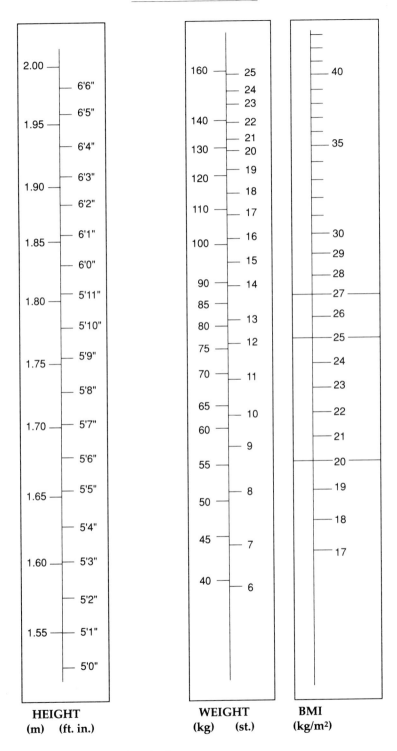

HEIGHT
(m)   (ft. in.)

WEIGHT
(kg)   (st.)

BMI
(kg/m²)

▲ *Body Mass Index Scale*

The further you go above 27 on the C scale, the more likely you are to face obesity and serious health problems such as heart disease, high blood pressure, arthritis, diabetes etc.

BMI between 25 and 27 is a caution zone. Watch your weight; you could easily swing into the danger zone.

BMI between 20 and 25 is a good range for most people. If you eat sensibly, your weight should not cause problems

BMI less than 20. You may be edging into the underweight category. Being seriously underweight can be equally dangerous for your health, leading to risks of anorexia nervosa and bulimia.

It is important to remember that there are physical features which cannot be altered, such as your bone structure. Just as you cannot change your height, you cannot attempt to alter the shape of your hips, shoulders etc. There is no point in grasping at false ideals. (After all, Marilyn Monroe was size 16!)

◆ ◆ ◆ ◆
SALUTE TO THE SUN SEQUENCE

This is a very ancient Yoga sequence which was traditionally practised at dawn. The sequence goes through a full range of stretching movements which should be carried out in a slow, continuous progression until you come right back to the original standing position.

Remember also that it is important to keep your breathing regular, doing your best to inhale and exhale evenly. This is best done before breakfast at an open window.

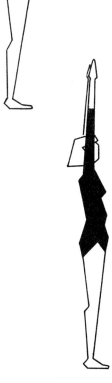

1. Standing. Feet together and palms together in front of you. Be aware of your posture and stand tall. Hold for 3.

2. Stretch the arms over the head and reach up as tall as you can. Feel the stretch along the chest and stomach. Hold for 3.

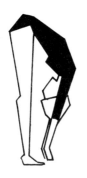

3. Bring the upper part of body forward and bend over. It doesn't matter if your hands don't touch the floor. Hold for 3.

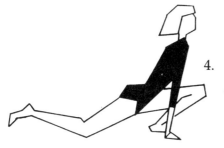

4. Bend both knees. Place the palms on the floor and push the right leg back. Keep the left knee bent up between the arms and stretch the chin up. Hold for 3.

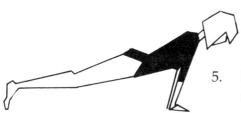

5. Bring both legs back. Keep the spine straight. Hold for 3.

6. Touch the knees, chest and chin on the floor. The bottom is in the air. Hold for 3.

7. Place the body flat on the floor and push up on the arms. Stretch the chin upwards towards the ceiling and keep the hips on the floor. Don't straighten out the elbows unless you find it comfortable. Hold for 3.

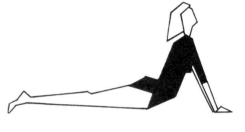

8. Bring the body up into an arch. Pull the tummy in. Heels on the floor if possible. Hold for 3.

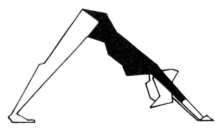

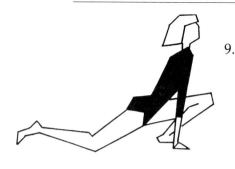

9. Bring the left leg forward. Place the knee between the arms. Stretch the right leg out behind you, hands on the floor, chin up. Hold for 3.

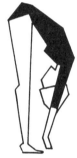

10. Bring the right leg forward and straighten out the legs. Relax your head and arms as you bend over. Hold for 3.

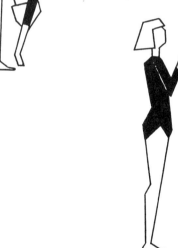

11. Slowly raise the upper part of the body, lifting the arms up over the head and stretch up as tall as you can. Hold for 3.

12. Bring the arms back down so that you come back to the starting position again. Hold for 3.

* Repeat the entire sequence 5 times. As this Salute to the Sun sequence becomes easier to do, you can increase the hold to a slow count of 5 or even up to 10.

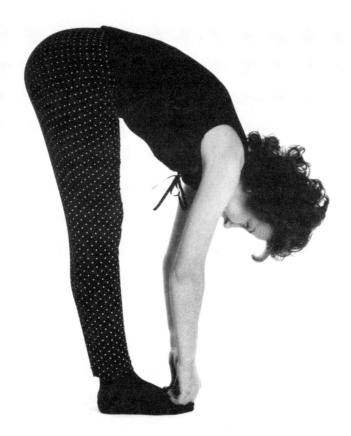

▲ *Don't strain when you bend over. It doesn't matter if your hands are not anywhere near the floor (Position 3).*

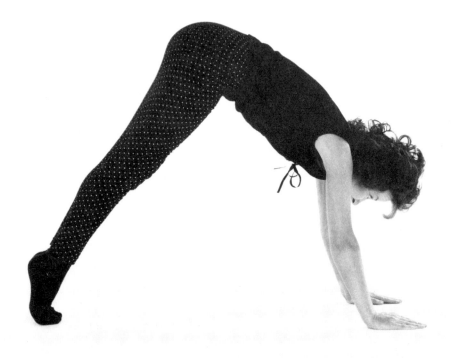

▲ *Jackknife up into this arched position. Come right up onto the toes and pull in the tummy. Wonderfully refreshing (Position 8).*

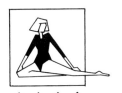

♦ ♦ ♦ ♦
5. A NEW OUTLOOK ON FOOD

♦ ♦ ♦ ♦
A Healthy Appetite

We can't stop loving food. So what we want to achieve in this chapter is a life-time appetite for good food. Instead of dwelling on all the highly calorific foods which everyone has to cut down on or cut out, you want to develop a taste for a healthy, balanced diet. The only way to lose weight is to eat three meals a day ... and nothing else.

If you are overweight, you need to cut down on calories without cutting out the essential nutrients, minerals and vitamins your body needs. By dieting or going without regular meals, you quickly set up an imbalance in these essential elements. That's the first step - never skip a meal. Be sure to eat breakfast, dinner and an evening meal.

Why not undergo this simple nutrition test to find out whether you are living on a balanced diet, whether you are getting the right nutrition, and, more than anything else, to check your dietary habits in general? Ask yourself the following questions.

♦ ♦ ♦ ♦
Nutrition Test

1. Do I ever skip meals?
2. Do I often consume cakes, biscuits, sweets or carbonated sweet drinks?
3. Do I have more than two alcoholic drinks per day?
4. Do I normally add salt to my food at the table?
5. Do I drink coffee or tea more than three times a day?

6. Do I add sugar to my coffee or tea?

7. Do I snack between meals?

8. Do I eat meat or meat products more than twice a day?

9. Do I cut out potatoes, bread, pasta or breakfast cereals?

10. Do I avoid vegetables, salads, fruit etc.

11. Do I omit seafood from my diet?

12. Do I eat desserts once or more each day?

Poor eating habits normally fall into these categories. There is excessive consumption of refined carbohydrates (cakes, sweets, products made with white flour or white sugar). Instead, you should be going for the more complex carbohydrates (fresh fruits, vegetables, whole grains).

Excessive consumption of fats is another category which can increase health risks and put on weight. Because animal protein contains a lot of hidden fat, it should also be watched.

◆ ◆ ◆ ◆
The 'Right Stuff'

What your body needs is a good balance of the three basics:

Carbohydrates + Fats + Protein

Carbohydrates, what we normally call starchy food and which for a long time was mistaken as fattening food, is in fact one of the essential elements of a healthy diet and weight control. A low carbohydrate diet causes instant and misleading weight loss. A rapid loss of water may cheer you up on the weighing scales, but it is a real swindle on the system.

Not only do you need sufficient carbohydrates such as bread, pasta and potatoes, as well as what you get from fruit and vegetables; you also need these nutrients three times a day. In addition, you should be going for whole wheat or whole grain products. Not only do they provide the necessary fibre; they also tend to be lower in calories and provide bulk which makes you eat less. With refined carbohydrates, what we normally call empty carbohydrates, you tend to need less chewing and tend to eat greater quantities.

Remember : Starchy food is filling and low in fats.

◆ ◆ ◆ ◆
Fats

Fat is a primary source of energy. Our bodies are extremely efficient in storing any fats which are not burned up through activity. Some storage of fats is essential to protect organs and to maintain body temperature as well as providing the body's necessary fatty acids.

There is a variety of fats: the obvious ones we find in butter, margarine, oil and the fat on meat. There are also the hidden fats in such foods as whole milk, crisps, peanuts, ice cream, cakes, biscuits etc. Try to avoid animal fats found in many products such as mayonnaise. Try using skimmed milk or products made on reduced fats. Go for leaner meat portions. Use the light varieties of oils and margarines.

Because of the incidence of heart disease now linked increasingly with the cholesterol found in animal fat products and eggs, these foods should be doubly watched.

◆ ◆ ◆ ◆
Protein

There are two varieties of protein: animal and vegetable protein, such as is found in lentils and beans etc. We need little more than two ounces of pure protein in a day. Any more will be converted into energy which is either used as fuel or stored as fat. Because animal protein is often couched in fat, it should be cut down. Instead, try going for other proteins stored in eggs (three a week maximum), milk products, grains and, of course, legumes (i.e. pulses and beans).

◆ ◆ ◆ ◆
Fine-tuning your eating habits

- Don't outlaw food. Cut back instead of cutting out. Cut back a little at a time and train yourself to eat smaller portions.
- Opt for low calorie substitutes - yogurt instead of cream, low fat milk instead of whole milk.
- Eat more starchy foods.
- Avoid all added sugar in your diet. Go for an apple instead of cake, or strawberries instead of strawberry flan.

- You will miss having lots of fats and sugar in your food, but your taste buds will soon adjust and begin to enjoy the crunch of raw carrots or celery instead. After a while, your instincts will form a preference for the natural sweetness of fruit over the cloying sweetness of cake.

- Train your taste buds with non-fattening flavourings such as lemon juice, herbs, spices, mustard and garlic.

- When eating out, go for poached fish, a small grilled steak, roast chicken (skin removed), pasta or a salad plate.

- Avoid alcohol. It's high in calories and low in nourishment.

◆ ◆ ◆ ◆
Organise Yourself

The best way of overcoming your bad eating habits is to take full control over your own diet. Don't be led by advertising or attractive packaging in the supermarket. Plan your shopping basket carefully. If you manage to come home without the old 'danger foods', then you have won half the battle. Remember the most valuable hint - never to go into a supermarket on an empty stomach.

Another good hint is to plan your meal by eating only what you place on the plate, then getting up and escaping out of the kitchen. Don't feel trapped by food. Develop other interests in life. Remember also that eating in front of the TV is one of the worst habits of all, principally because you are not really aware of what or how much you're eating.

- Cut out salt. It causes the body to retain fluid and contributes to high blood pressure.

- Cut right down on coffee, tea and chocolate. They all contain caffeine which can lower the blood sugar and ends up making you feel hungry.

- Cut out fizzy drinks. Most soft drinks contain sugar and caffeine. Most diet drinks contain salt.

- Eat no more than three meals a day. If you want to have a snack in between, go for healthy foods like yogurt, fruit, vegetables or whole grain bread.

- Eat only when hungry. Always sit down to a meal. Eat slowly, chew thoroughly and make sure that you eat in a calm atmosphere.

- Let nothing put you off! Encourage yourself. Don't drop your efforts because of one mistake. There's no hurry. Time is on your side.

◆ ◆ ◆ ◆
THE SPHINX SEQUENCE

Anyone who carries excess weight in the stomach area will undoubtedly very soon experience back trouble of one sort or another. The muscles in the stomach do a valuable job in supporting the spine. With a pot belly, spare tyre or slack stomach muscles, you can automatically force an enormous burden on the back.

The Sphinx Sequence is specially designed to strengthen the back and to make the muscles supporting the back strong and supple. A strong back will help to get rid of any aches and pains after a long day. If you're one of those who has never suffered from back trouble, then keep it that way by doing the Sphinx Sequence regularly.

As you go through the poses of the sequence, keep in mind the image of the catlike Sphinx creature resting on top of an ancient Egyptian tomb.

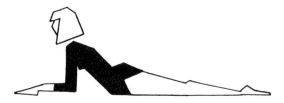

1. Lie on your stomach with your elbows on the floor directly beneath your head. Palms flat on the floor. Raise your head up as high as you can and stretch back without removing the hands or the elbows from the floor. Hold for 3. Come back to the starting position.

2. Without moving the elbows or the hands, turn the head and the upper part of the body to the left, attempting to look at your feet behind you. Hold for 3. Come back to starting position.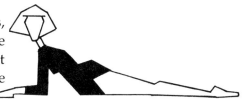

3. Turn the head and upper body to the right. Hold for 3 and come back to the starting position.

4. Raise the hands and the legs up into the air. They may only lift an inch off the floor. Remember to *keep them straight.* Hold for 3. Then lower again.

5. Remaining flat on your stomach, place the legs well apart and bend your right knee up. Catch hold of the foot with your right hand. Hold for 3. Lower the leg and straighten it out.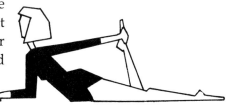

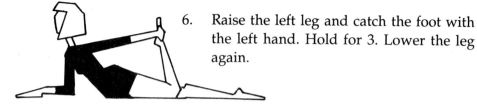

6. Raise the left leg and catch the foot with the left hand. Hold for 3. Lower the leg again.

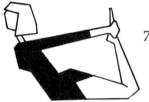

7. Raise both legs and catch hold of both feet with both hands. Hold for 3. Lower both legs.

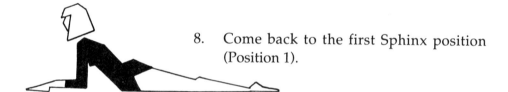

8. Come back to the first Sphinx position (Position 1).

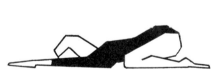

9. Keeping your hands on the floor, bring your body back so that you end up sitting on your heels. Put your head down on the floor. Stretch out as long as you can with your arms.

   Enjoy the comfortable feeling of this final position for a while before you repeat the sequence again.

*Repeat the entire sequence 5 times. As with the other sequences, increase the hold to a slow count of 5 or even 10.

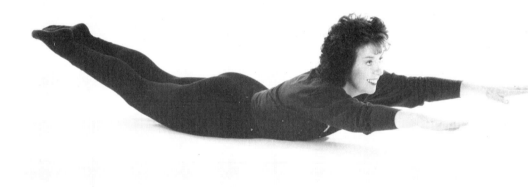

▲ *Marvellous for strengthening the back (Position 4).*

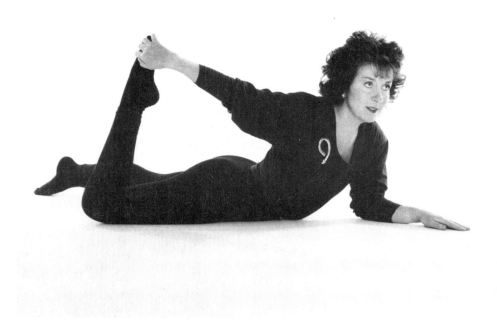

▲ *This pose is easier if you place the legs well apart (Position 5).*

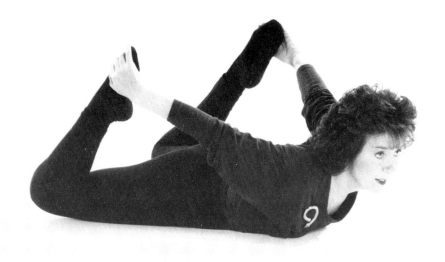

▲ *Easier than it looks (Position 7).*

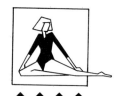

◆◆◆◆
6. STEPPING UP THE PACE

◆◆◆◆
Into the Fast Lane

Once a day, or at least three times a week, you should feel your own heart beating fast. Not because you've been looking at a Hitchcock film on TV, but because you've asked your body to increase the effort. Why? Principally because you want to increase the capacity of the heart and lungs. Secondly, because you don't want any loose calories being stored up as fat. And more important still, you want to be healthy.

Getting yourself slightly out of breath three times a week is absolutely essential. In the past few years there has been an inordinate emphasis on cardiovascular fitness: running, jogging, aerobics, circuit training etc. In other words, you had to get a real sweat going and be seen darting along the road with a purple face before you could be redeemed and pass for normal.

Experts today are once again pushing the case for moderation. Running a mile uses up exactly the same amount of calories as walking a mile. So why not walk? If you like running, well and good. But the experts are now stressing moderation in exercise. By walking a mile, you spend perhaps ten minutes more than you would running the same distance. But walking is just as good.

◆◆◆◆
Your Beating Heart

Think of your body like a machine in which your heart, a large muscle, pumps blood around the system. In simple terms, when you exert the body by running or walking, the blood delivers oxygen and glucose to the body's muscles. At the same time, it performs a waste disposal operation by carrying back CO_2 out through the lungs. In principle, that is why you breathe in and out at a faster rate when exercising and why you get out of breath when you're unfit. If you are not fit, the heart and lung system lacks the capacity to do the job efficiently.

Everyone knows the feeling of stiff, maybe aching, muscles after the first exercise routine. A brief explanation of this is that the blood has not been able to deal with the excess waste (lactic acid) in the muscles. A good reason to keep up the exercise from there on. What happens when you increase the work load on your muscles is that the body quite naturally demands more oxygen. Consequently, as the oxygen is carried throughout your body, it improves the condition of your blood vessels, unclogs fatty deposits on the arteries, burns energy (i.e. calories) and greatly improves the expansion capacity of the lungs.

This is what is called aerobic exercise. As you become fitter and your lung capacity improves, so does the ability to endure aerobic activity for longer periods. It also increases the body's capacity to restore the health of its tissues and organs. You won't feel the muscles aching any more, you'll have an honest appetite and you'll have a lot more energy.

Exercise generates energy. It's obvious: the more you exercise, the more your body wants to exercise.

◆ ◆ ◆ ◆
Fitness Test

The first thing to do is to find out how fit you are. There are various elaborate methods available to get what's called your VO2 max, in other words, your body's oxygen uptake; and by extension your body's ability to recover. A simple test you can perform on your own is by walking for five minutes at three miles per hour (twenty steps every ten seconds). At the end of five minutes, take your pulse for one minute.

Place two or three fingers (not thumb) on the pulse of your wrist. Count the pulse you feel in a minute. If your heart rate is over 100, you are out of shape. You need aerobic fitness. Go for a complete medical check-up and consult your doctor on choosing an aerobic programme.

◆ ◆ ◆ ◆
Choosing Exercise

- Find an exercise routine you can live with. No point in starting something like tennis unless you really like it.
- Be realistic. Don't be hard on yourself. Don't rush into a failure by taking on an advanced aerobics class.
- Work your way up to fitness. Take your time. After three weeks, you should begin to feel the benefits.
- Choose a continuous aerobic activity: walking, swimming, cycling, dancing or competitive games.

◆ ◆ ◆ ◆
Exercise Myths

- Exercise does not give you a ravenous appetite. After three weeks, your body will adapt while your appetite normalises.
- Exercise does not exhaust you. It gives you a healthy, relaxed, tired feeling, a good sleep at night and ultimately a lot more energy.

◆ ◆ ◆ ◆
Metabolism

One of the key effects of increased aerobic activity as part of an overall exercise plan is the benefit from a raised metabolic rate. This is the rate at which your body burns up fat ... all-important to weight watchers. Not only is this metabolic performance better during exercise, but it's now proved that the metabolic rate remains higher long after you've finished exercising.

◆ ◆ ◆ ◆
Yoga

Yoga adds to all of this as a perfect complement by warming up and cooling down the muscles after an aerobic workout. One or two sequences before and after your brisk walk or your game of squash

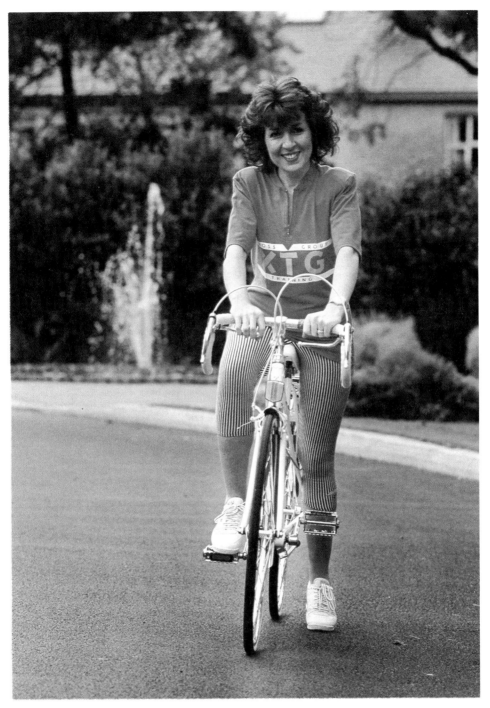

▲ *Stepping up the pace ... on the way in to RTE.*

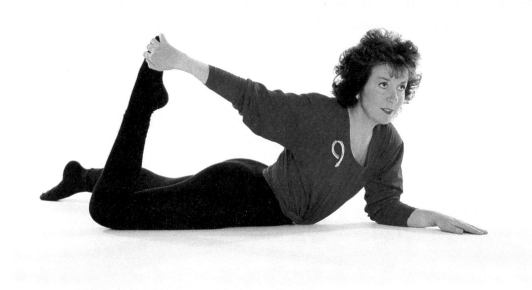

▲ *Yoga is like a password for relaxation (The Sphinx Sequence).*

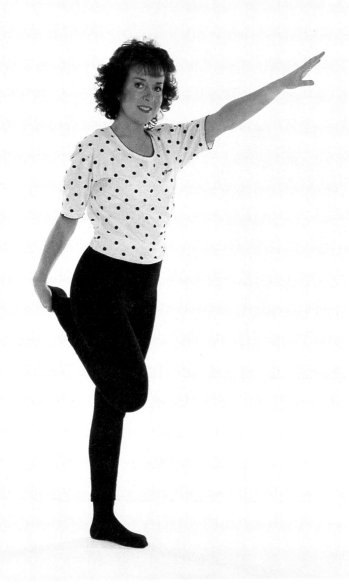

▲ *Balancing calms the mind and improves the posture (The Stork Sequence).*

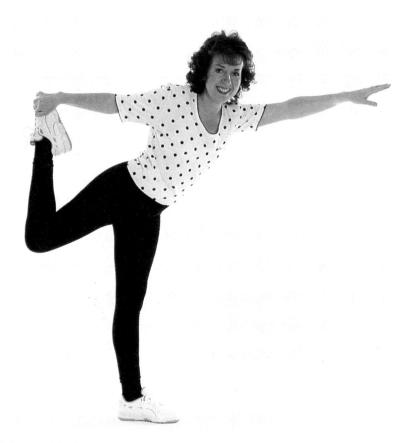

▲ *A pair of shoes might keep you from wobbling (The Stork Sequence).*

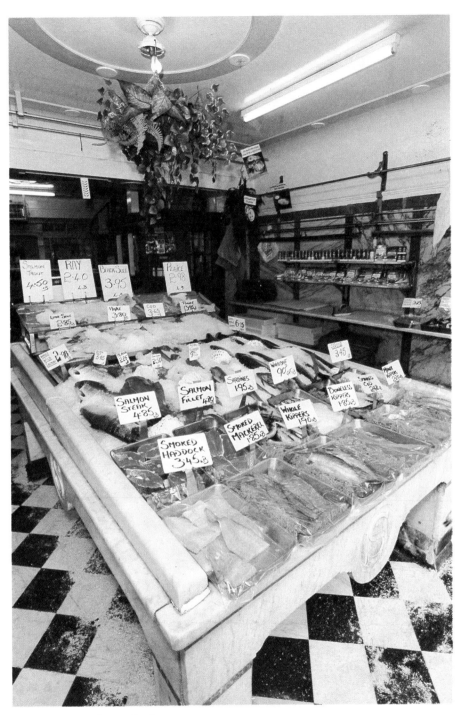

▲ *Seafood is brain food.*

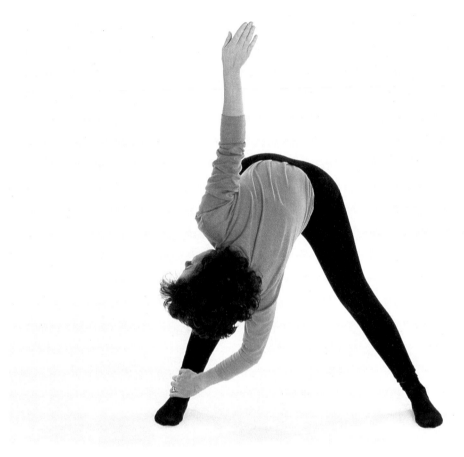

▲ *Releasing trapped energy (The Warrior Sequence).*

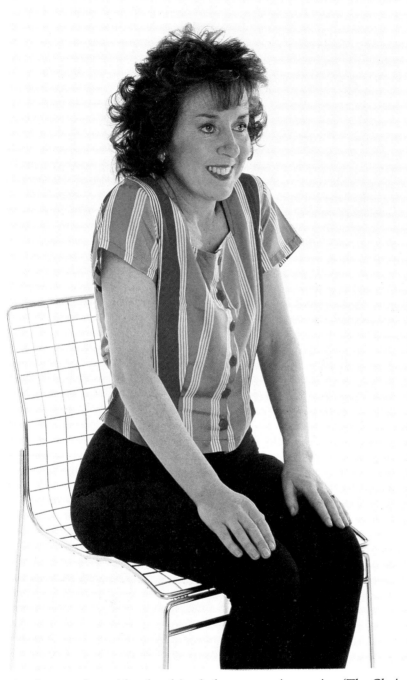

▲ *Get together with a few friends for an exercise session (The Chair Sequence).*

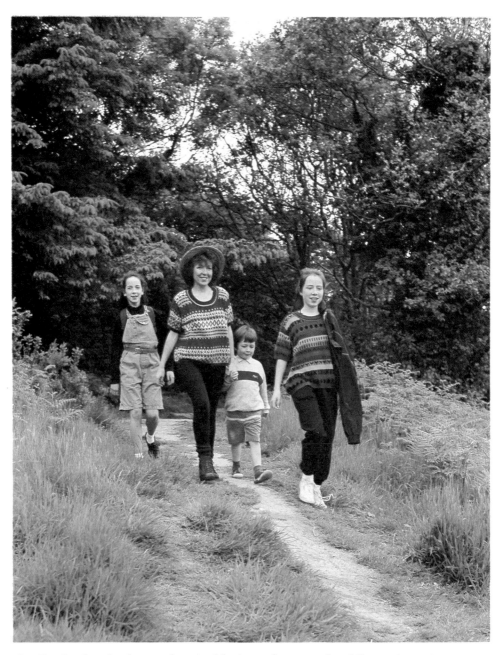

▲ *Getting lost in the woods ... and losing a few pounds while you're at it.*

will stretch and prepare your muscles. You will also find that, when the body is warmed up after a walk, the Yoga sequence is that bit more enjoyable and relaxing.

◆◆◆◆
Walking

As far as I'm concerned, walking is one of the most perfect aerobic workouts you can get. It has been put in the shade for too long by jogging, running and aerobic dance classes. Like Yoga, walking is now making a worldwide comeback as one of the most accessible, safe, cheap and enjoyable forms of exercise.

Walking, or what they now call power walking, burns up energy at a substantial rate, equal to running or swimming. You will burn around 300 calories in a thirty minute run. A forty minute brisk walk will do the same and is obviously a lot safer all round, putting less stress on the heart and less pressure on the body in general.

Walking doesn't mean a stroll around the block. It means pushing yourself at a good, brisk pace, the speed at which armies march.

Find out the distances involved and do a twenty to forty minute walk, three times a week. Many people I know have begun to do this every day, walking in the local park or out in the country.

One of the most positive benefits of walking is the rhythmic cadence which the repeated footfalls set up. This has a calming effect on your mind. You start talking to yourself and remove yourself from the stress in your life. Walking does not require any equipment; a pair of good shoes at most. You may progress to hillwalking, in which case you might like to invest in a pair of sturdy boots.

If you have easy access to walking routes such as the Wicklow Way, you can't avoid being fit. Holidaymaking has also moved away from the idea of lying on the beach to the more healthy breaks organised around walking holidays, whether in the Black Stairs, the Pyrenees or the Hindu Kush. If you really want a spectacular walk, why not try the five mile cliff walk along the Giant's Causeway.

◆ ◆ ◆
Cycling

One of my own favourite ways of getting in to the 'Live at 3' studios is on my bike. Cycling is one of the best forms of cardiovascular exercise, whether you stay put on an exercise bike or whether you like to see the scenery passing at the same time. The benefits of cycling go mainly to the legs and heart.

Mind you, cycling is one of the toughest sports, so it's important to map out a spin that suits you. One thing to remember about cycling is that if you have back problems, you should take it easy and make sure you don't remain bent over the handlebars for too long in one stretch. Like swimming, cycling is a weight supportive exercise with little stress on joints. You'll find this a very comfortable way of getting into regular cardiovascular fitness.

◆ ◆ ◆
Addiction

You can become addicted to exercise. Because of the production of endorphins, the brain's natural opiates, the ability to suppress pain is raised through energetic exercise. So people who work out regularly experience a great overall feeling of well-being during and after exercise. It has been described as an exercise 'high'. It's a healthy addiction. Not only does it help to reduce the dependence on other addictions - smoking, coffee, alcohol etc. - it also increases that powerful, rewarding feeling of success and calm satisfaction.

Walking, cycling and Yoga together make the best all-round combination of both cardiovascular and stretch exercise which is easy to assimilate into almost any lifestyle. The combination will have a lasting effect and give you complete health.

◆◆◆◆
THE WARRIOR SEQUENCE

The Warrior Sequence is a very invigorating series of poses which tones and stretches the entire body. Working especially on the thigh and calf muscles, the sequence also gives shape to the waist, bottom and arms.

Move in slow motion from one pose to the other. If you find that you are not as supple as you would like to be, don't worry. You'll be amazed at how quickly the body becomes strong and supple.

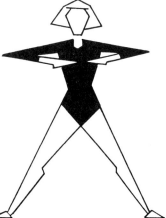

1. Stand tall. Feet well apart. Stomach and buttocks in. Shoulders rolled down and back. Place the tips of the fingers together in front of the body, elbows bent. Hold for 3.

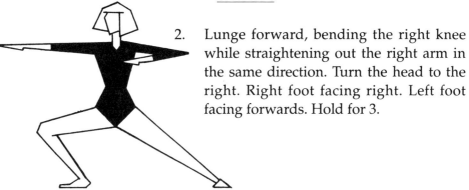

2. Lunge forward, bending the right knee while straightening out the right arm in the same direction. Turn the head to the right. Right foot facing right. Left foot facing forwards. Hold for 3.

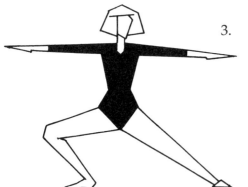

3. Without moving the lower part of the body, stretch the left arm out. At the same time, turn the head around to the left. Hold for 3. Bring the head back.

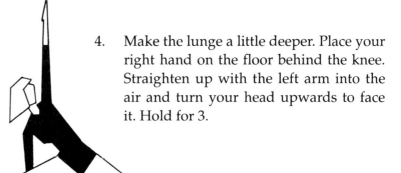

4. Make the lunge a little deeper. Place your right hand on the floor behind the knee. Straighten up with the left arm into the air and turn your head upwards to face it. Hold for 3.

5. Remain in the same position and put both hands on the floor on either side of your right foot. Turn your left foot towards the right. Lunge down as low as you can. Hold for 3.

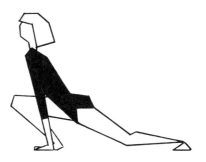

6. Keeping your right hand on the floor, slowly stretch your left arm up into the air. Hold for 3.

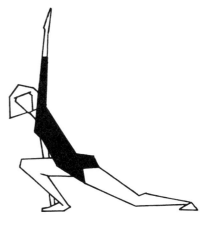

7. Return your left arm. Stretch your right arm into the air as in position 6. Hold for 3.

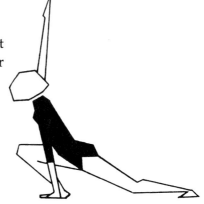

8. Return your right arm. Putting both hands on your right calf, gently pull your head towards the knee. If you can straighten out with the right leg, that's great ... if not it doesn't matter. Hold for 3.

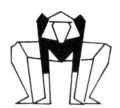

9. Walk your hands from the side around to the front. Make sure the knees are bent. Relax into it. Hold for 3.

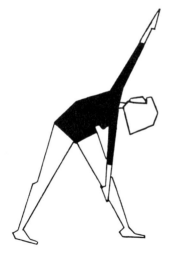

10. In the bent-over position, gently straighten the legs and put your right hand on your left thigh. If you are a little more flexible, you may be able to put it on the knee, the calf or even the ankle ... remember, there's no rush. Very smoothly, raise the left arm into the air and look up towards it. Hold for 3.

11. Do exactly the same with the right leg and left hand. Hold for 3.

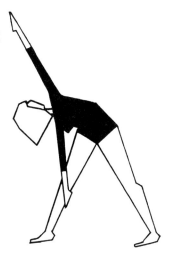

12. Slowly, slowly raise yourself until you are standing in position 1.

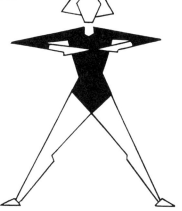

* As soon as you have finished, repeat the entire sequence with the left leg. Work up to going through the Warrior 5 times on either side. If you wish, increase the hold for up to a slow count of 5 or even 10.

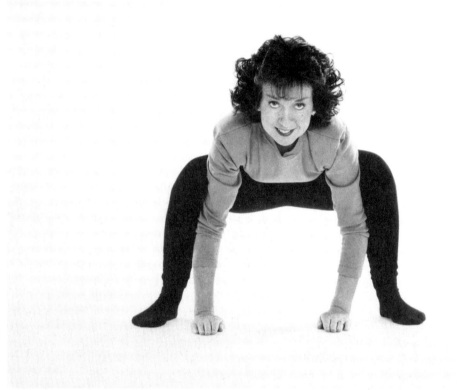

▲ *Keeping your knees bent protects the lower back (Position 9).*

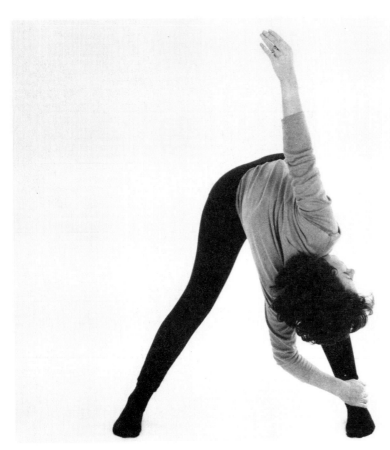

▲ *If you can't reach down to the ankle, then put your hand on your calf or knee instead. Remember, there's no rush (Position 10).*

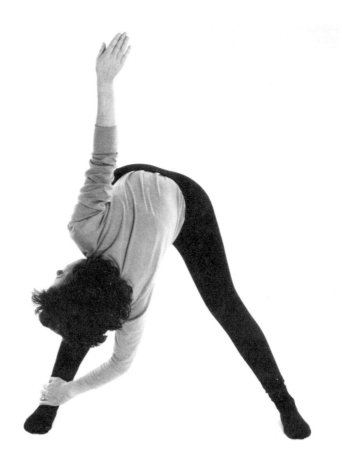

▲ *Raising the arm into the air should be done very slowly to avoid straining the back (Position 11).*

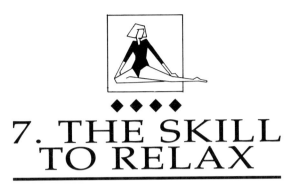

7. THE SKILL TO RELAX

Why are so many people turning back to Yoga and stretch exercises right now? For one thing, the superior benefits of relaxation which are associated with Yoga have been proven over and over again. Yoga is like a password for relaxation. Certainly, the people I know who have practised Yoga over the years have kept their calm and relaxed attitudes. They know how to relax. What's more, their bodies relax automatically, without thinking.

Without this skill, many people admit that their bodies would instinctively go in the opposite direction. Like relaxation, tension is purely a habit which is inclined to build up. Why do we get tense? The answer is that our bodies are designed to react that way. We are designed to react with tension; a perfectly natural response to danger. The trouble starts when we perceive imaginary danger; when we over-react and keep up our guard all the time.

◆ ◆ ◆ ◆
Trapped Energy

It is useful to think of tension in the body as trapped energy. All that energy you would use to run away or get out of danger gets trapped every time you don't spring into action. You only have to watch a tense person lift a cup to see how we often invest far too much effort in an activity that really should be much easier. The same goes for our bodies in general. So often, we quite naturally spend too much effort on minor daily activities such as gripping the phone or the steering wheel of a car.

The fact is that we allow our anxieties to magnify without giving them the chance to wind down. We can become besieged by our personal environment (i.e. work, family life, social situations). Besieged by our own personal troubles, we often quite simply forget to relax.

One of the best things about Yoga and the flexibility you can achieve through these sequences is that your muscles will learn to release that trapped energy. The muscles will be in better condition and the body will call upon its own resources, what's known as the 'relaxation response', to deal with anxieties. Tension will be released quite naturally.

◆ ◆ ◆ ◆
What is stress?

Stress is what makes us react. Anything in our environment or personal life which arouses our natural human responses can be called stress. We tend to think of stress as a bad word. In fact it's neither bad nor good - it's neutral. Everything we react to or get excited about is stress. And quite simply, if you don't react well to good news, if your body can't wind down after excitement, then you'll hardly expect to come off well with bad news either. We tend to forget that the body has an inbuilt response to stress which should instantaneously wind down when we are out of danger.

Perhaps you've often wondered why so many people go quite voluntarily to see horror movies and subject themselves to a high degree of stress. It's stress without consequence. Afterwards, you can wind down, say to yourself it was just a movie and forget it. That is how we need to relax in our daily life too. Once every day, we need to wind down completely. That is exactly what Yoga and positive relaxation do.

◆ ◆ ◆ ◆
The Stress Test

Before you ask yourself the following questions, remember that when the body receives the stress signal, it reacts with the following responses. The muscles tense up and get ready for action. The heart beats faster. You breathe faster and more erratically. The blood rushes to the head to make you more alert. Digestion is postponed and your mouth goes dry. Over a prolonged period, without release, this causes a dramatic increase in tension. If the tension doesn't wind down quickly then there is something wrong and you need to develop the skill to relax.

Are you too tense? Ask yourself the following questions.

- Do you jump at unexpected noises?
- Do you often get headaches or pains in the neck, shoulders or back?
- Do you find yourself in hunched or tense postures?
- Do you sleep badly and wake up feeling tired?
- Do you easily get angry or impatient?
- Do you have an inability to express emotion or enjoy yourself?
- Do you get obsessed by worries?
- Do you resort to bad habits like overeating, smoking or drinking too much?

◆ ◆ ◆ ◆
How to Relax

The best time to start thinking about relaxing is after you have done a thorough Yoga session, when the muscles of the whole body have been exercised. Once the body is relaxed, the mind will also begin to relax.

Your daily relaxation session should last twenty minutes at least. If you are very tense, you may find shorter periods more effective in the beginning. You may also find that you become drowsy at the first sensation of pure relaxation. No harm. Many people find themselves falling asleep, an indication that it is working for you. But the basic idea is to try and relax consciously.

Comfort is very important. Lie down on the floor or sit in a comfortable chair. Make sure that your back and neck are well supported. On the floor, place a slim cushion under your head. You should be warm. If you like, you can cover yourself with a blanket.

Start off with some calm, rhythmic breathing. Breathe as noisily as you can so that you become aware of yourself inhaling and exhaling. Blow the breath out, pulling the tummy in as you do so. Slowly, begin to inhale. As you take air into the lungs, your tummy should begin to lift up. The ribcage expands and then finally the chest.

This very act of conscious and calm breathing will trigger off a relaxing sensation throughout the body. Because we focus on the peaceful to-and-fro motion of each breath, our tense and menacing thoughts will begin to disappear. It's almost like lying on a beach listening to the constant surf breaking and receding, forwards and backwards again and again. We thrive on repetition. If the room is silent, even the rhythm of your breath will sound just like the sea.

Visualise that image in your mind. The idea is to slow down the breathing to a smooth, even rhythm. So often our breathing remains rapid and shallow. Keep up this slow breathing for a short while. When you get more practice, you will be able to go into this calm breathing during your Yoga sequences.

◆ ◆ ◆ ◆
Give yourself a talking to

There is nothing wrong with talking to yourself. In fact, it happens to be one of the most positive ways of systematically relaxing every part of the body. As you are sitting or lying down, try focusing on different areas and telling yourself that they are becoming relaxed.

'... I feel calm and relaxed... My forehead is smooth and free from tension... My eyes are still and comfortably closed... I will allow my jaw to relax... My tongue is relaxed in the centre of the mouth... There is no tension in my face.'

'... I have pulled my shoulders down and back... My neck is free and loose... There is no tension in my arms and hands... I have let go of all the tightness in my stomach and my breathing is calm and rhythmic... My legs feel heavy and my whole body is beginning to sink down... The pressure has disappeared...'

Continue with this systematic method until you have worked your way down through the entire body. Then you can concentrate once again on your deep breathing, focusing on the image of the waves coming in and going back out again.

◆ ◆ ◆ ◆
THE STORK SEQUENCE

The Stork Sequence could be described as relaxation in action. In each of the poses of this sequence, balance, poise and posture are exercised and improved. However, it's extremely important that you relax as much as possible while going through the Stork. If you hold your breath and allow the body to become tense, you'll find it much harder to keep your balance.

Balancing poses force you to concentrate; they calm the mind and improve the posture. Practitioners of Yoga will talk about an improvement in strength, agility and co-ordination.

Hold on to a table or chair for balance if you find the poses difficult. Take your time and be patient. If you find yourself hopping and wobbling all over the place, don't give up! After you've practised for a few weeks, you'll be amazed at how much better your balance has become.

1. Stand tall. Become aware of your posture. Shoulders down. Stomach and buttocks in. With your feet slightly apart, exhale noisily and deeply. As you begin to inhale, slowly raise the arms out to the side and right up over the head. At the same time, come up onto your toes. Exhale, lowering the arms and coming back down onto the feet. Repeat this 3 times. Be aware of your breathing throughout the entire sequence.

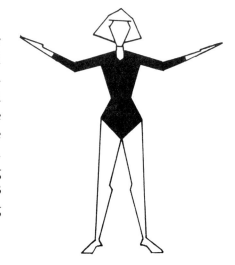

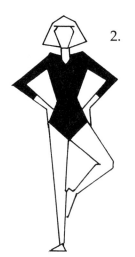

2. Place your hands on the hips. Lift your left foot up until it rests on the right calf. Hold for 3.

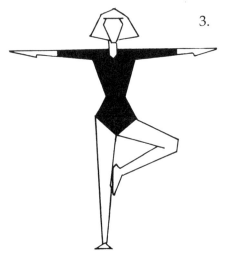

3. Without letting your left foot touch the floor, smoothly slide it up to the knee. Raise your arms out to the side. Hold for 3.

4. Remain standing. With the right hand, place the left foot on top of the right thigh. Push the left knee back to prevent the foot from sliding. Slowly bring your hands up until they meet up over the head. If you find this pose too difficult, then remain in position 2 or 3. Hold for 3. Lower your left foot to the floor.

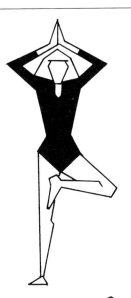

5. Bend the right knee up behind you and catch hold of it with your right hand. Hold onto the wall with your left hand if you find you are losing your balance. Hold for 3.

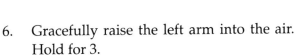

6. Gracefully raise the left arm into the air. Hold for 3.

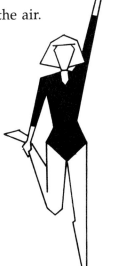

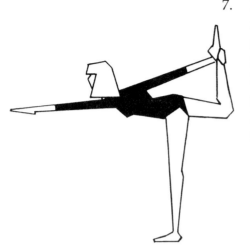

7. Now we'll try balance in motion! Remain in position 6. Begin to extend your left arm out in front of you. At the same time, stretch your right leg out behind. Do this all very slowly. Remember to relax and breathe in and out deeply. Hold for 3. Lower your right leg, but do this smoothly, with control.

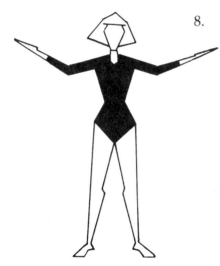

8. Place your feet slightly apart. Breathe out. As you begin to inhale deeply, lift your arms up at either side of the body and come up onto your toes. Exhale, lowering the arms back down and coming down onto the feet again.

* Repeat the entire sequence 3 times with each leg.

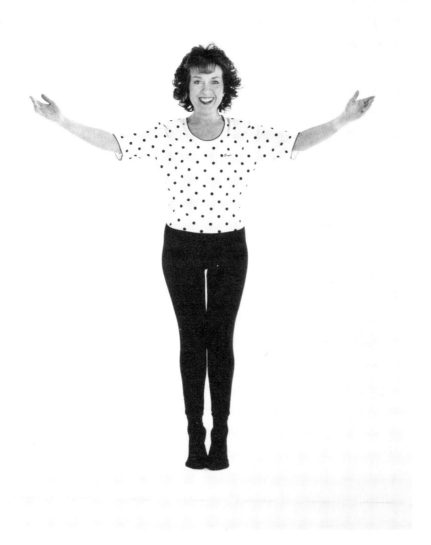

▲ *Come right up onto your toes as you inhale deeply (Position 1).*

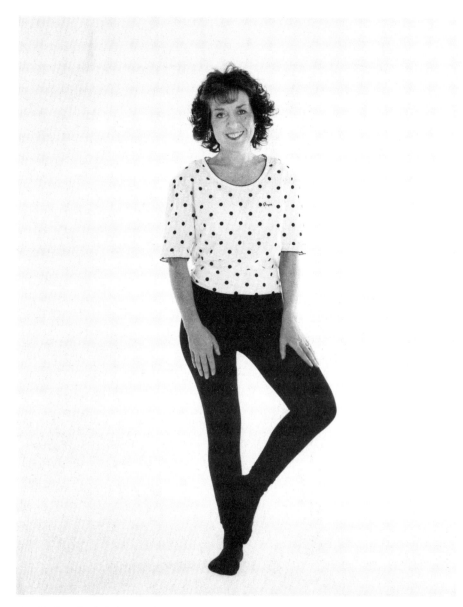

▲ *Raise the left leg and place it along the right thigh. Hold on to a chair for balance if you wish (Position 2).*

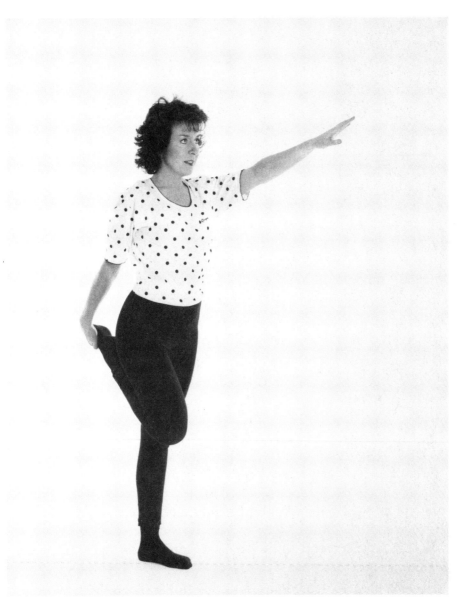

▲ *Move slowly and breathe evenly. Balancing is good for your concentration (Position 6).*

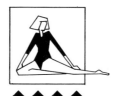

8. NEVER TOO OLD

No matter what age you are, it is never too late to start a new, more active lifestyle. If you have had an active life, so much the better. But it is important to realise that from the age of forty onwards, the body goes into a very slow decline. Nothing to be alarmed about. This natural ageing process can be made comfortable and painless with a moderate amount of exercise and, of course, healthy eating.

It is perfectly possible to feel and look wonderful right up to the age of eighty. One may also feel youthful and energetic by taking part in life and refusing to hang up your limbs. If you want to take part in this new emancipated age where senior citizens lead a full and enjoyable life, then why not take on a safe and easy exercise routine?

◆◆◆◆
Changes

First of all, you can't ignore the facts. Age is recorded in the body with a number of clear features. After the age of forty, loss of muscle strength and the redistribution of body fat causes subtle changes in the shape of the body. Men tend to develop an abdominal bulge, whereas women tend to become fat around the waist, hips and bottom.

It's not just the fact that we notice our hair going grey or the wrinkles appearing; there are subtle changes happening in the whole body. The bones, arteries and tissues deteriorate. The body becomes stiff and the joints lose their range of movement. Much of this cannot be avoided. What can be avoided, however, is a rapid premature ageing.

By exercising and becoming active even in a moderate way, you can prolong your interest in and zest for life. Remember that the process is a gradual one. A lot has to do with your personality. If you remain physically active, you will also remain mentally active. A lot can be done to slow down the effects of getting old by improving your posture, keeping to a regular exercise programme, singing, dancing and enjoying life. If you haven't picked up the walking buzz, then there's no better time to start.

Your doctor will tell you exactly how much you can take on. It's important that you go for this consultation, especially if you suffer from a bad back, arthritis, rheumatism or have a heart problem. No matter what kind of physical shape you are in, there is always some kind of exercise routine that you can undertake. However, it has to be a routine that is tailor-made for you and your body. Otherwise you may end up doing more harm than good.

◆ ◆ ◆ ◆
Yoga for Senior Citizens

Yoga, of course, is an ideal form of exercise for all of us, no matter what age. It is especially suited to those of increasing years because of the slow-motion, no-strain approach to movement. It is also very effective in improving the circulation and warming up the body. Because Yoga movements greatly improve flexibility in the joints and limbs, you will feel great relief if you suffer from arthritis and rheumatism (again, check with the doctor).

To derive maximum benefit from your exercise routine, keep to a regular programme and do your exercises at the same time each day. Before a meal is the ideal time. For a change, you could try putting music to your exercise session to make it more enjoyable. No harm as well to keep in mind a good aerobic exercise such as brisk walking. Because the rate of recovery is not as rapid in older years, it is important to slow down or even stop if you find that you are becoming tired. Take it easy. The principle is frequent, light exercising.

A good diet is equally important in keeping up both your energy and your spirit. Not only is it important to avoid too much cholesterol for those who have heart ailments; it is also good to avoid salt, especially if you suffer from high blood pressure. Many older people begin to lose their appetite, others gain appetite. So it's necessary to take account of all this at retirement age.

Retirement is the perfect time to become involved in all those activities which may have eluded you up until then. If you can opt for outdoor, energetic pursuits, then so much the better. With a regular Yoga routine, you'll have a whale of a retirement and lead a full life.

◆ ◆ ◆ ◆
THE CHAIR SEQUENCE

The good news about exercising in the chair is that it's just as effective as other forms of exercise. And don't for one minute think that it's an easy way out. Your chair routine can be as strenuous or as gentle as you want to make it. This sequence is aimed mostly at those who may not be as energetic as they used to be, or those who are incapacitated in some way. It's a good idea, of course, to get the doctor's approval first.

Choose a sturdy chair for this sequence. Make sure that it stands firmly and that the floor is not slippery. Wear loose, comfortable clothing and don't forget to slip off the shoes. Why not do this routine with a few friends? It makes exercising a lot more fun. Begin each routine by doing some slow-motion neck rolls and shoulder rolls.

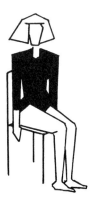

1. Sit on your straight-backed chair. Your back should be long and your shoulders down and back. Keep the tummy pulled in throughout each movement.

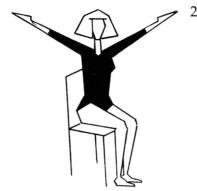

2.   We begin by taking in a complete breath. Do this a number of times with your arms raised, similar to the Stork Sequence. As you inhale, lift the arms up into the air at either side of the body. Exhale, lowering the arms. Repeat this 3 times.

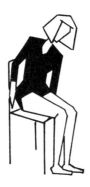

3.   With the arms relaxed by your side and the feet firmly planted on the floor, slowly relax your body to one side. Make sure that you are leaning to the side only, not forwards. You don't want to put a strain on the back. Relax the head over also. Hold for 3 in each position. Repeat 3 times on each side.

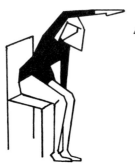

4.   Now we'll stretch the waist a little more. Lift up your right arm and bend over to the left. You will feel a greater pull along the side of the body. Remember, if it hurts, then lift yourself into a position that's more comfortable. Hold for 3 and repeat 3 times on each side.

5. Why not work that waist a little more? Raise both arms into the air and clasp them together. As you bend over to the left side, make sure that you protect the back by leaning to the side and not forward. Make sure too that all your movements are performed slowly and gracefully. Hold for 3 and repeat 3 times on each side.

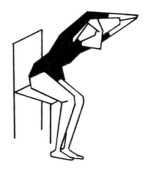

6. Now, let's tone and firm the legs. Arms by your side, raise the right leg off the floor and straighten it. Flex the right foot by bending it back and hold for 3. Then, without jerking, point the toes in the opposite direction. Hold for 3. Flex and point the toes 3 times. Repeat with the left leg.

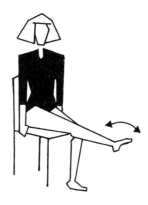

7. Circle the ankles of each foot 3 times in either direction.

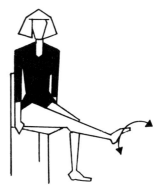

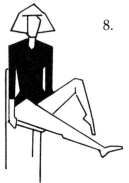

8. Sitting a bit closer to the edge of the chair, lift both legs an inch or two off the floor. Keep them straight. Cycle the legs one after the other. Repeat these movements 10 times. This cycling movement tones the stomach muscles and strengthens the legs.

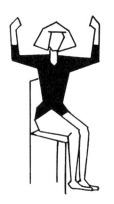

9. Sit up tall in your chair. Stretch the arms out on either side. To firm up the biceps, bend and straighten the arms. Repeat 10 times.

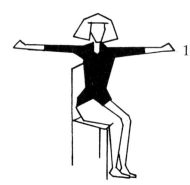

10. Keep the arms stretched out on either side. Clench and stretch the hands. This exercise is wonderful for improving the circulation and strengthening the arms. Repeat this 10 times.

11. Bend over. To firm up the triceps muscles which run under the arm, lift the arms up behind you. Straighten the arms and slowly bend them. Repeat this 10 times.

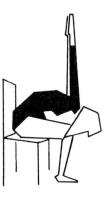

12. Now relax the arms and head as you remain in that bent-over position. If your hands touch the floor, that's great. If not, it doesn't matter in the slightest bit. As with all our exercises, it's very important that you never strain. Hold for a count of 10. Sit up gradually.

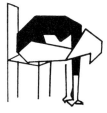

There are many other exercises you can do in the chair. You could also try standing and holding onto the chair and raising and lowering your legs individually. Try also bending and straightening the legs and coming up and down on the toes. Repeat 10 times.

Give yourself time to relax afterwards. If you wish, repeat the entire sequence 3 times.

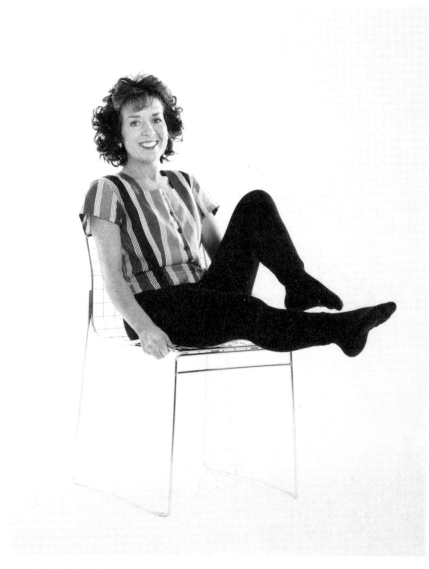

▲ *Cycling in the chair is a wonderful tummy toner (Position 8).*

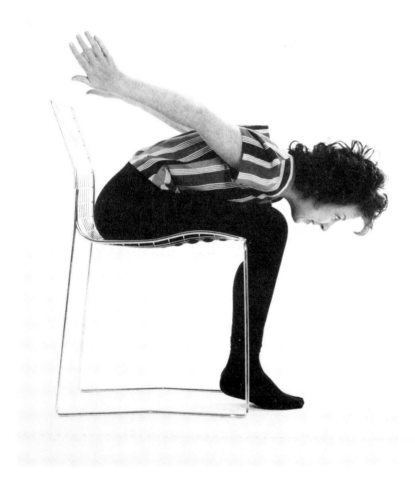

▲ *Straighten and slowly bend the arms to firm up the underarm muscles (Position 11).*

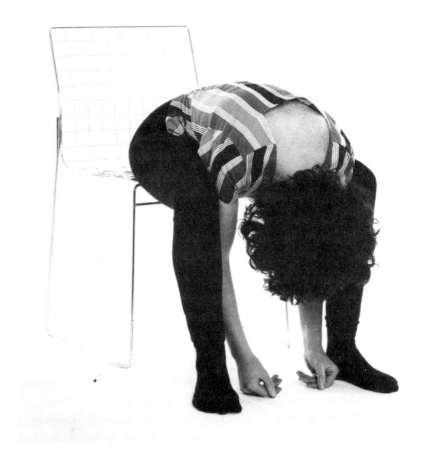

▲ *Bending over in this position is incredibly relaxing and refreshing (Position 12).*